The Single Person's Guide to Surviving Shoulder Surgery

ISBN: 9798697569894 (print)

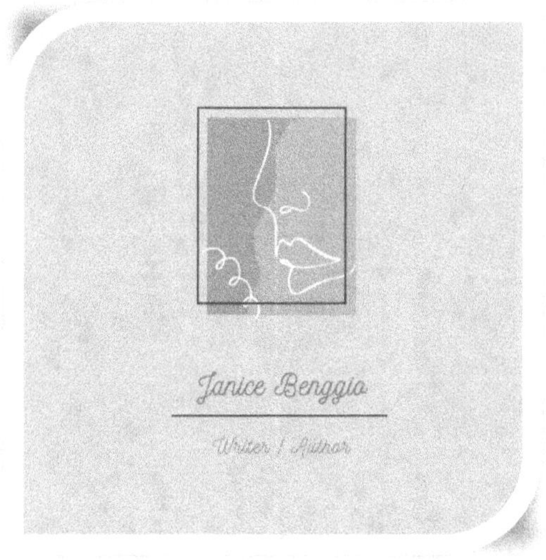

Special thanks is given to the Veterans Administration Health System for the care they provided throughout this journey. This is a picture of the Panama City Beach Florida VA Outpatient Facility, where my care is coordinated. This facility was recently recognized as having the best patient satisfaction scores in the entire VA Health System, with a perfect 100% satisfaction rating. The caregivers there have been outstanding with me, and it's clear that they have the same level of professionalism for all their patients. Thank you, VA Healthcare System!

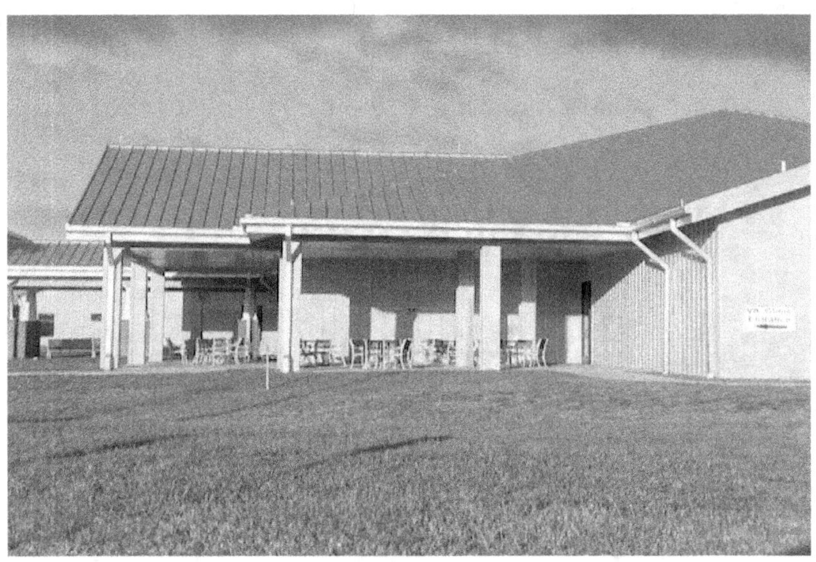

Dedication

This book is dedicated to friends, family, and co-workers who offered advice, assistance, or simply words of encouragement. I especially thank Jamie Shepard, my co-worker, who had the same surgery I had on both shoulders within a year. Her support and encouragement was the voice of true experience, mixed with her witty way of saying it would be okay. At one point she said together we made almost one complete worker in the office. Also, Mom and Kathy McCurdy were invaluable to drive me around, keep me company, and do anything else I needed. Thank you all.

Table of Contents

This is a guide, especially for singles and those who live alone and have shoulder surgery. People with partners can benefit, too, but single people are generally very independent and used to taking care of themselves with ease, so they don't always make the best patients. That's why I'm sharing this information from my experience, so you can also remain as independent as possible after surgery. Get someone to stay with you for the first day or two if you can, as those are the most difficult days.

It's not always "old people" that have shoulder problems, as athletes and clumsy younger people find themselves in this predicament, too. Anyone that does repetitive work that taxes the shoulder can find themselves in pain and may take some hints from this guide as they give the injured arm and shoulder a break. I'm not a medical expert, nor am I a physical therapist. I am someone who dealt with a shoulder injury for a year and almost gave up when physical therapy stopped working. That's when I knew that the only fix was a surgical repair. I'm not one of those people that will keep hoping something will get better, because I look for the fix, and an orthopedic surgeon was my answer.

There are some unique challenges when it comes to using a single hand and arm, often the non-dominant one, and not having another human in the house to assist after surgery. Pets might keep us company, but they certainly can't use their paws to help with these challenges. Preparation is the key to having a successful recovery. Healthcare providers will give you their general instructions, but there were many points that I've learned from my own experience. Being resourceful has been helpful, and it also takes a bit of determination to get through this with as little dependence as possible on pain meds and other people. Friends and family who have also had this surgery gave some helpful hints, and I've learned a few tricks myself, so here they are to hopefully help you have a more trouble-free journey.

You may not remember much about your ride home from surgery, and that's not a bad thing. Hopefully, you won't need the emesis bag (for throwing up), but you'll undoubtedly have a friend or relative driving you, and they will understand the situation.

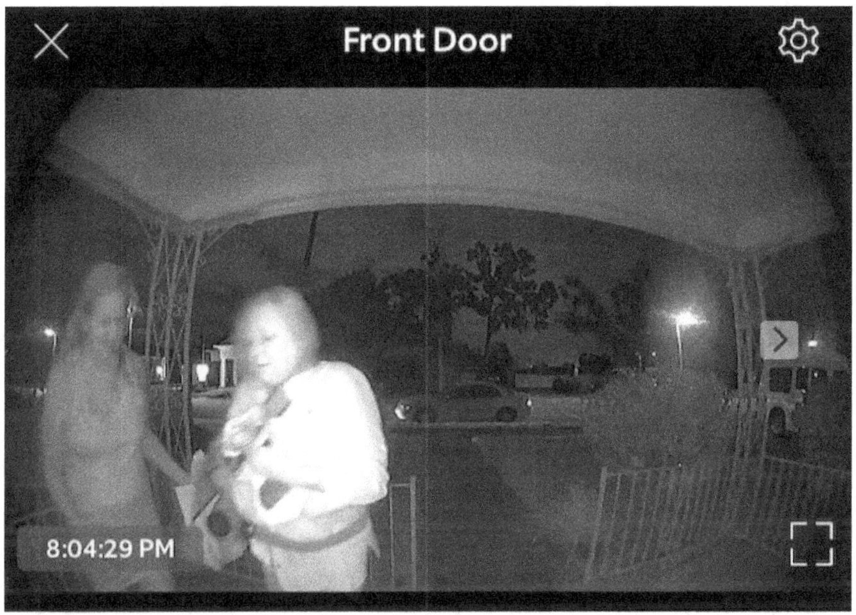

I later found that my security camera captured that moment I got home, desperately clutching my vomit-bag from the hospital. My friend, Kathy, was very patient to wait for me to have the stability to step in the front door. I was in a very foggy state and have little memory of this time period.

This is me about 12 hours after coming home from surgery. I look like I've been hit by a train, and I guess I talked my mother into handing me the computer. I recall being frustrated with one-fingered typing, so I didn't do much for a few days. Notice that lump on my shoulder, which were bandages of gauze. You'll later hear about button-up shirts, which were definitely good to have for the first few days.

The best advice for the first couple of days is to follow the surgeon's instructions exactly. They should be written instructions that were either given to prior to surgery or as you were leaving surgery. You'll want to have your pain prescription filled and have some simple snacks and water or other beverage handy. Don't let pain catch up to you during these first hours, as it's more difficult to deal with it once it hits. Again, just follow directions or have your caretaker (if you're lucky enough to have one stay with you initially) understand and guide you. The effects of anesthesia are usually present for at least 24 hours, so be comfortable and rest during this time.

Pain Control

At the time of this writing, it has been just less than three weeks from surgery, and pain is less than what I expected. I had a nerve block during the procedure so that kept me from experiencing pain for the first couple of days. It wore off and I did have some pain for a few days. Everyone is different, but my pain was tolerable and relieved either by the occasional prescription pain med or an over-the-counter NSAID.

I'll offer a word of caution about using prescription pain meds, which may not be a problem for most, but it is for me. When I'm hopped up on everything that is given during surgery and then take pain meds at home, I think I feel good and am in control. I'm not in great control, and I've realized this pattern from prior surgeries. I once reunited with an old boyfriend while under the influence. This was years ago. I had questioned how he knew I was in the hospital, and he said I called and told him. I somehow had the presence of mind to find his number, but would not have done that in my right mind. Therefore, for my shoulder surgery I warned my co-workers in advance that I sometimes say or do things I shouldn't and to please forgive me if that should happen this time. As much as I tried to control myself, I still made a few poor decisions (the ones I remember) during the first few days.

I sent a group text message to my co-workers about wanting to go buy a bunch of flowerpots and needing a ride to the beach to get them, but I meant to send that message to a friend. I was in no shape to go shopping or do any planting. M y co-workers ignored me, and my friend (who got the same message later) didn't take me to buy them. They all made correct decisions. My other thing was buying a bunch of expensive knives. True, I needed some knives, but I probably shouldn't have spent that much at once. At least I've crossed the loopy threshold and haven't heard about other things I did under the influence. There's a reason we're told to not drive, make major decisions, etc. while taking pain meds. This is another good reason to have someone stay with you for the first couple of days.

I typically know how to spell, how to type, and how to send messages to the correct person, but this went to my co-workers. Also, I usually take time to compare prices and get the best deal. This deal was expensive, but they've turned out to be great!

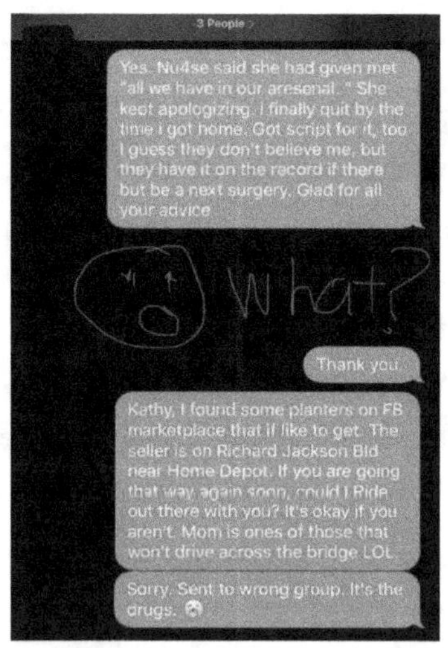

Most prescription pain medications have a few side effects that could be annoying, such as having a dry mouth and constipation. Keep plenty of water handy to sip all day and night, as it helps with both of those problems. It might also be helpful to get some stool softener tablets before surgery and take them as needed during the time you take the prescription pain medication.

The most pain came from the sling and accompanying "pillow," which keeps the arm abducted. It never seemed to fit correctly, and I think that one of the straps was missing a ring or something. I'm awful at reading diagrams, so it's likely my fault that I took it apart and put it back together wrong. I used a soft washcloth around the neck strap to keep from rubbing my skin raw. I also placed a hand towel at the bottom of the sling, because it was too large and held my hand too low. This helped lift my arm slightly.

Ice packs help relieve pain. I thought I had an ice bag but could not find it when I got home. I found that plastic freezer bags are perfect for holding several ice cubes. I place it on my shoulder to relieve pain for 10-20 minutes, and the baggie can be used repeatedly during recovery.

If you're like I am, the pain that led to the decision to have surgery has already forced you to make several changes before your surgery. Sometimes they are so subtle that you don't notice them. It could be as simple as not using the injured hand and arm as much and relying more than usual on the non-injured side. Consequently, you're probably somewhat ambidextrous by now. That will be a distinctive advantage in your recovery. In fact, it can be beneficial long after recovery, unless you overdo that side and injure it – don't do that!

Food and Drinks

We all have to eat, so plan out how you will accomplish this before your surgery. I cooked meals before surgery that could be frozen and heated up as I wanted them. Make sure that you have fairly small portions because you might not be too hungry during recovery and also because you don't want to lift things that are heavy. Containers should be lightweight, easy to grasp, and easy to open. Keep a small pair of scissors handy to open bags. Friends and family may offer to bring food to you, and you should take them up on it. People often want to help and don't know how, and this is one way that they can definitely help you.

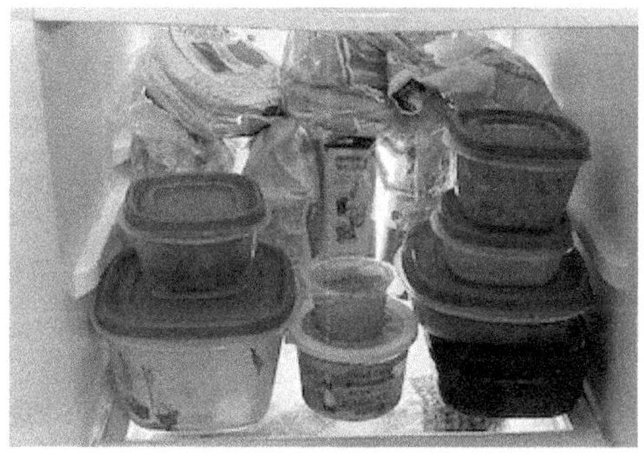

These are a few pre-made foods that I could quickly grab without much trouble.

When you do feel well enough to cook, keep in mind that you'll be limited with how much you can do with one hand. One example was that chopping veggies was hazardous (sharp knife and not good control). Using gadgets like food processors and blenders is helpful, as long as they are already handy and you don't have to lift them. Even if you like preparing your own fresh food, this is a time that having some already-prepared foods can save time and frustration.

Opening bottles and jars (even medicine) can be almost impossible with one hand. I had bought an electric bottle and jar opener years ago and rarely used it. However, it has been a very valuable tool during my recovery. Otherwise there are certain items I would not have been able to open items if it had not been for this gadget. You can often find these at thrift stores for very little money. If you don't need them later, you can always donate or pass them along to someone who could use them. If you have medicine in a "blister pack," you may want to open them before the surgery and put them in a container that's easier to open. Another thing to be aware of is child-proof containers, which can be impossible to open after surgery. Prepare how to deal with that pre-surgery.

Your surgeon may have specific recommendations for food and drinks, but mine suggested some vitamin and mineral supplements, along with milk. I don't care for milk but can tolerate it with cereal. That worked out well, because I like high-fiber cereals, which has the needed feature of keeping the gut working.

Personal hygiene will truly be challenging for a while. The surgeon will let you know when it's safe to shower. I was lucky in that I could start showering after only 3 days. Even so, using one hand makes it difficult to reach all the areas that you want. Be sure to take care of major grooming chores before surgery, including hair coloring and haircuts, waxing, tweezing, shaving, manicures, pedicures, and so forth. It could be several weeks before you get to do all of those again, or at least with any degree of comfort. Of course, you could pay someone to do these for you, but you may not feel like doing them, and you won't be able to drive for a while.

Even underarm deodorant may be a little difficult. If you're used to using solid deodorant, you might consider changing to a spray for a short time. I found that if I hold a solid deodorant with the good hand, I can probably get the product under the surgical side if I can move my arm out a little. But, it's tricky the other way around. I had to hold the deodorant, bend and twist in hopes of getting it under the non-surgical arm. Good luck, and just make sure no one's watching or listening to you swearing as you do this dance. My instructions were to keep the sling on all the time except for when I was doing physical therapy or personal grooming, so I delight in these moments of temporary freedom, even if they come with a little pain.

I found that small washcloths are much better than large, thick ones that are difficult to handle. A soap bar might be easier to use than liquid soap with a scrubby. Shampooing won't be the same, either. One friend suggested using a cheap hairbrush to help distribute the shampoo on the scalp and scrub it well. Having a handheld shower is essential for rinsing yourself and the shower.

Wiping one's nether regions with the non-dominant hand might not be so easy, and the toilet paper holder might be located on the side of your surgical arm. If you can put a roll of paper in a more convenient location, you'll be thankful that you don't have to contort too much to reach it. I have a bidet, the kind that installs easily under the toilet seat. This has been a wonderful way to stay clean down there, especially when one hand is incapacitated. The problem is that the button to activate it is on the surgical side. Hence, that toilet paper being handy was important.

Dental hygiene is very important, as bad dental hygiene can sometimes lead to medical problems. Therefore, you may want to have your routine dental cleaning scheduled shortly before you have your surgery. A good way to keep your mouth clean is to use an electric or battery-powered toothbrush and/or a water flosser. This is especially true if it's your dominant hand is out of commission. If you don't have those, try practicing brushing your teeth with the weak hand before your surgery so you can get the hang of it. Also, for some reason I seem to get toothpaste on my shirt more now, so don't get dressed in anything nice before brushing.

Combing or brushing your hair with one hand feels strange, but it can be done. One thing I could not figure out was how to put my hair in a ponytail or a clip, because I couldn't use only one hand to do it. I was able to do a side ponytail after a couple of weeks, and it kept hair out of my face but looked ragged. Don't worry about makeup and jewelry or trying to look good, because you probably won't.

As to clothes, you may find it very difficult to get your clothes on and off while being gentle with the surgical arm. You might want to practice this before your surgery to get an idea of the best ways to do it. It had to watch videos to find a method that worked for me. One of my friends suggested I get some button-up men's shirts before surgery, because they are easier to get on and off than pull-over shirts for the first couple of post-op weeks. She was absolutely right with this suggestion. I went to a thrift store outlet and found clothing that was sold by the pound. I got dozen shirts for a couple of bucks. They were actually very good shirts, in great condition, and I can give them to someone once I've recovered. Another reason these shirts are useful is that you will not be able to wear a bra for a while. Your shoulder will be swollen, and you may have stitches close to the bra straps . Also, it is physically hard to put on and take off the bra only one-handed or with limited use of the other hand. Eventually, I learned how to do it by lying it on the bed and doing the surgical arm first, fastening in front, and slowly sliding it around and into place.

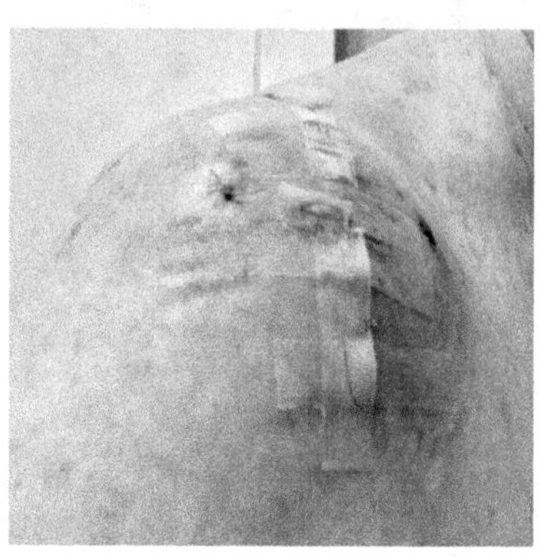

Clothing has to navigate around this, and you don't want to

disturb or irritate it at all.

I had to go to a party during my recovery, and I wore a dress that zips in the back. This would not have been possible except that my mother came over and zipped my dress. I freaked out when she brought me home and left, and I realized I was still in the dress. I'm a little claustrophobic but knew that if all else failed, I could cut it off with scissors. I didn't want to call her to come back just to unzip me, so I struggled with my decent hand to reach the zipper and worked it down a little at a time. It took an inordinate amount of time and energy to get out of this dress, so I will never make that mistake again. Simple clothing is definitely best while you recover. Slip on shoes are great. I definitely love my flip-flops, and I live in Florida, so it's pretty easy to dress casually here. I'm really not sure how to handle it if you have surgery in the winter and live someplace where you need lots of warm clothing. I guess the best thing would be to stay in the house while you recover. I don't know how to live in a cold climate anytime of the year, surgery or not.

       This photo was not
the birthday party
referenced, as I don't have a
picture of being in that
zipped up dress. This was a
little later. It was a pullover
dress with a large neckline,
which was easy to put on
and take off. The necklace
had a magnetic clasp, which
allowed me to put it on and
take it off easily at the front.
There was no way to do
anything with my hair, other than combing it with my non-dominant
hand. The humidity didn't help. Both my shoes and my watch band
were secured with Velcro® closures, making it easy to adjust with
one hand. I removed the "pillows" from the sling, even though it was
a little early to do that. I didn't feel like being out of the house much,
but it actually boosted my spirits to be around some friends for a
quick birthday gathering.

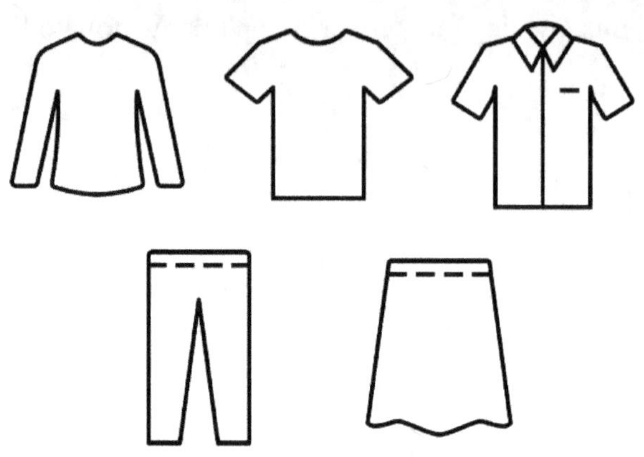

Plan in advance what you can easily wear

Around the House

Going to Work

Shopping

Medical and Other Appointments

Physical Therapy

Social Events

Consider ease of access to put on and take off, pockets, access to or covering of surgical wound, security and safety, weight of fabric and accessories, and of course, comfort. Elastic waisted pants and skirts will be much easier to wear than anything with buttons, snaps, zippers, and hooks.

Sleeping can be a challenge, and you probably will not be comfortable in your bed for a while. Ideally you should have a recliner that you can operate with your non-surgical hand. For example, if you had surgery on the right shoulder, it would be helpful to have a recliner with the control on the left side. My reclining loveseat was ideal, because I had a table and lamp on the left side, and could put other items within handy reach on the right cushion. This was my bed for more than a week. A friend used a bed buddy pillow for sleeping, but I found that to be more trouble than it was worth. When I did try to use my bed, it took a while to find a comfortable position, and I had to stay on my back so I didn't move my arm. Get lots of pillows so you can set up your nest to be comfy. Don't be surprised if you wake up with pain or from just being uncomfortable. It's good if you're able to take a nap during the day in case you didn't sleep well during the night.

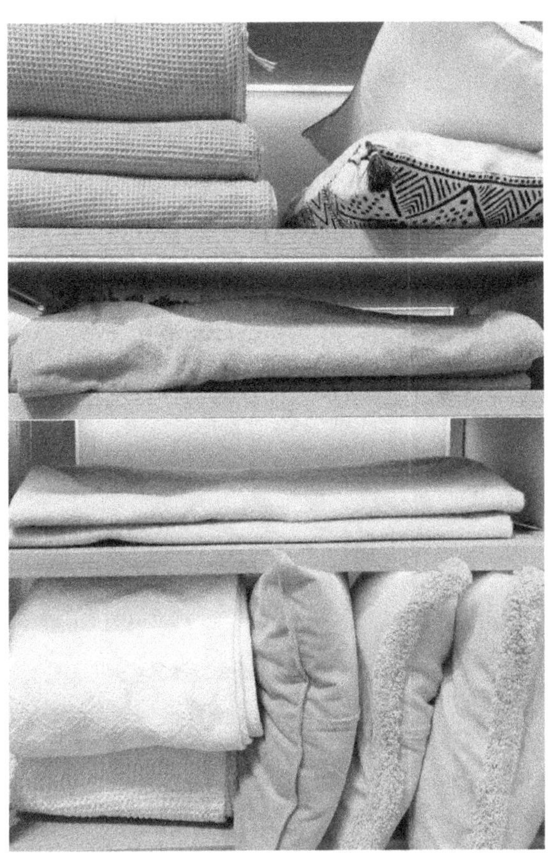

Whether you sleep on a recliner, your bed, or something else, you'll want to have some pillows, blankets, or towels to help prop you in a comfortable position that will keep your surgical arm as still and comfortable as possible.

Photo by Taisiia Shestopal on Unsplash

Be sure to arrange for someone to drive you to your physical therapy and doctor appointments until you are cleared to drive by your doctor. If you can't find a person to do it, look at public transportation or ride sharing apps. If you have a friend or relative do this for you, be sure to buy gas for them or offer some token of appreciation for their trouble and expense. It's a good idea to get some cash before your surgery for tips and other small expenses you might encounter.

NO DRIVING – CONSIDER PUBLIC TRANSPORTATION OR A FRIEND'S HELP

You may be tempted to drive, but don't do it until cleared by the doctor. Even if you're not on pain meds and feel you could do it,

it will take a while to get sufficient range of motion to safely
maneuver all the steps needed to safely be on the road, not just for
yourself but for everyone else on the road. Your short, little dinosaur
arm will not cooperate and stretch as far as needed, so just don't do it.

My work and much of my life involves using a keyboard. It is slow and tedious to use one hand and even one finger to type. I found a dictation program on the internet that lets me dictate, and I copy take that information into another application as needed. This is very helpful, especially for large amounts of typing. You'll definitely need to review it and make corrections before considering it final.

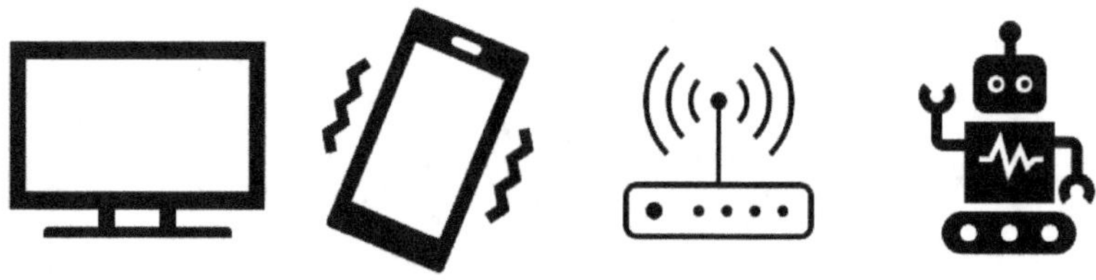

If you have a smart home device (Google Home, Alexa, etc.), you can ask them questions rather than trying to reach for a computer for phone. Sometimes I'd wake up in the middle of the night on my recliner in the living room and wonder about the time. My watch and phone were charging in another room, but I asked my handy electronic assistant, who cheerfully gave me the answers I wanted. They are also good for placing calls to your contacts if you misplace your phone or need to call and can't get to your phone. They can even call your phone to help you find it, which is a realistic expectation when you're on pain meds.

If your shoulder had been painful for a while, you may have already gotten a robot vacuum cleaner. It is very difficult to sweep, mop, or vacuum using only one arm, although it can be done, just not as well as you probably did before your injury and surgery. I use a push-button dispenser for dish soap, but it is not always convenient when holding a dish and trying to push the button at the same time with the same hand. Therefore, I keep a bottle of dish detergent next to the faucet, making it much easier to pour detergent on dishes and then wash them with one hand and a scrubber. The dishwasher is another good source of help, but if you live alone, you sometimes don't have enough dishes to justify using it. Give yourself a break during recovery and use it.

To help around the house, I bought a grabber that has a trigger handle at one end and a claw at the other end to reach small items that are not easily accessible otherwise. Honestly, it has not been that helpful, probably because I had already moved most things to better reach them. I had already bought a suction cup grab bar for the shower and a shower stool, which are definitely helpful during recovery. I don't use a shower mat, but it might be something to consider so that you maintain stability after your surgery. Drying off and wrapping your wet hair in a towel will not be easy, but you'll figure it out. If you don't, you can drip dry.

Laundry is a chore that does not take a vacation even though you may not feel like doing it. You'll do yourself a favor by having small, lightweight bottles of detergent and fabric softener. I moved my laundry basket from the bedroom closet to the laundry room to put my dirty clothes. That way I didn't have to lift the basket and move it to the washer. I could still do the laundry with one hand; it just took longer than normal. I was not able to fold my clothes as perfectly as I would like. I didn't care.

Clean your house very well just before surgery and there's a good chance it will stay in good shape while recovering. If not, offer a friend some cash to come over and help tidy it. As mentioned, you may be able to do many of the chores yourself with one hand, but sweeping and mopping isn't easy to do one-handed.

Safety is very important. Little things that seem insignificant could have a big impact. For example, if you have throw rugs, they might enhance the look of the room, but they could also cause you to stumble and fall. The last thing you need after shoulder surgery is to injure yourself. Look around for any potential safety hazards and remedy them before surgery.

If you don't have all your bills set-up to be paid automatically, make sure that you take care of all bill payments for the first month of recuperation. Taking pain meds or just not feeling well could cause you to forget to pay them, so it's better to do this in advance as much as is possible.

31

Pets need continuity of care, no matter how incapacitated you might be. Make a plan of how this will be done, particularly if you can't do it yourself. You might have someone come to assist, let your pet have a sleepover at a friend's place, or consider boarding them for a few days. I found that even some simple things were difficult. My cat likes a type of food that has a foil top that must be peeled back to open. I had no strength to open it for a few days. Thankfully, he had other foods, but even the canned foods were a harder to open than I'd expected. In retrospect, I could have used some cleaned out salsa jars to put several containers of food in, and then open that with more ease.

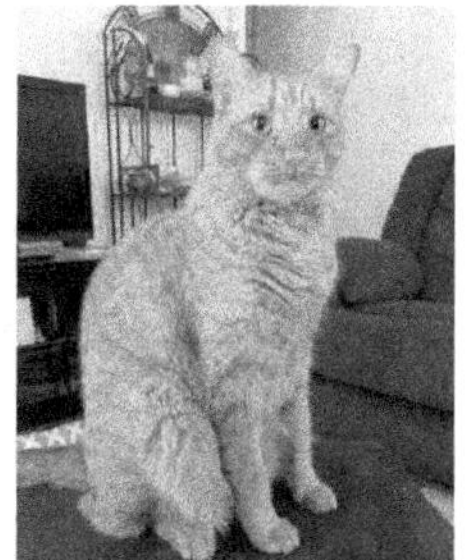

You probably won't be able to pick-up your pet for a while, but hopefully you'll find other ways to show affection to your pet. Some pets need to be walked or taken outside, but can you handle it one-handed? Some of them sense your condition and won't mind, but if you have an emotionally needy pet, find a surrogate to help.

Other

There are other things that I did not cover, but my advice is to go around the house before you have surgery and look for anything that could be moved or rearranged to make life easier. You could also try doing things with your non-surgical arm to see how it works. Doing this can alert you to changes that need to be done in advance.

I'm definitely not the best patient, because I'm way too impatient with progress. But knowing the end result will be much less pain with improved range of motion are what push me to reach my goals. I wish you the very best experience in your recovery.

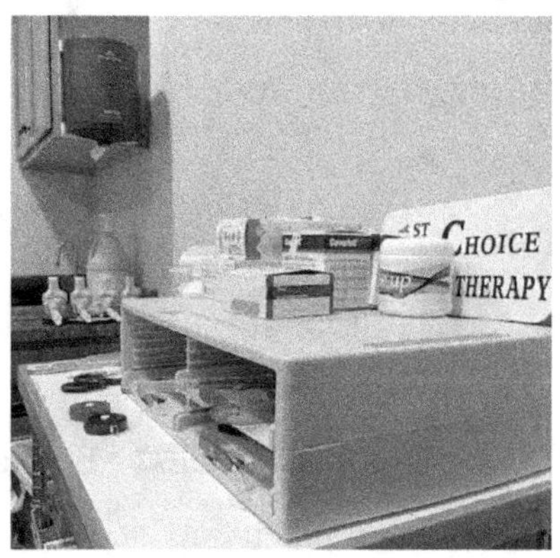

Janice Wells Benggio is a native Floridian who has worked half her career in the legal and judicial field and the other half in hospital administration (medical staff services and project management), with an MBA in healthcare management. She has been a consultant in the latter part of her career but has always found time to write as an outlet to express ideas, opinions, and information, or sometimes to spin a story from her imagination.

Janice's life has been full of varied experiences and diverse friends, all of which she credits for making her the inquisitive person she is today, always seeking to learn more, especially from and about people she meets. She currently lives in her hometown of Panama City, Florida, in the Northwestern Panhandle, returning from living a decade in Southeastern Florida (Broward County). She has two adult sons and their wonderful wives, along with three (and a fourth to arrive soon) beautiful granddaughters. Her only roommate is a large ginger kitty named PJ, who is completely spoiled, and she wouldn't have it any other way.